"My Journey"

By

Sabrina Renee Washington-Powell

ISBN-10 150564190X ISBN -13 9781505641905

CONTENTS

CHAPTERS

ACKNOWLEDGMENTS

THIS BOOK IS BEING DEDICATED TO MY MOTHER. SHE HAS BEEN THERE FOR ME THROUGH THICK AND THIN. SHE HAS HELPED GUIDE ME IN SITUATIONS THROUGHOUT MY LIFE AND HAS BEEN FAITHFUL IN PRAYING FOR ME IN EVERY CHALLENGE THAT I HAVE FACED. SHE NEVER JUDGED ME NOR HAS SHE MADE ME FEEL INADEQUATE. IT IS BECAUSE OF MY MOTHER'S LOVE THAT I DEVELOPED FAITH AND TRUST IN THE LORD. IT'S GOD WHO HAS GIVEN ME THE STRENGTH, WISDOM AND THE COURAGE TO SIT DOWN AND WRITE MY FEELINGS, THOUGHTS, and BEHAVIORS. ALSO TO WRITE THIS STORY ABOUT ONE WOMAN'S STRUGGLE WITH HER HEALTH, RELATIONSHIPS AND CHILDHOOD.

I WOULD ALSO LIKE TO THANK ALL OF MY TRUE
FRIENDS AND FAMILY MEMBERS FOR HANGING IN
THERE WITH ME DURING THE TIME I WAS WRITING
THE BOOK. YOU'RE ENCOURAGEMENT AND
PRAYERS MEAN SO MUCH TO ME.

A SPECIAL THANKS GOES OUT TO MY SISTER-IN-LAW WHO
EDITED MY MANUSCRIPT. I APPRECIATE YOU AND ALL
THE TIME YOU SPENT PROOFREADING THE BOOK. THANK
YOU TO MY FAMILY AND FRIENDS WHO CAME TO MY AIDE
WHEN I WAS STRUGGLING. YOU ALL KNOW WHO YOU
ARE. I LOVE YOU ALL SO VERY MUCH. WORDS CAN'T
EXPRESS MY APRRECIATION FOR YOUR LOVE AND
SUPPORT. THANK YOU JESUS FOR LISTENING, ANSWERING
MY PRAYERS, AND GUIDING ME AS I MAKE THIS JOURNEY
AND ONCE AGAIN TAKE ON A NEW CHALLENGE OF
WRITING THIS BOOK.

CHAPTER 1

ONE STEP AT A TIME

This is a story about a woman whose name is Sunnie Davis. She told me her story about the way she grew up and requested that I write this book for her. This book is written for men and women of different walks of life, races, ethnicities, lifestyles and socio-economic backgrounds. This is a book about relationships: good, toxic, bad, and ugly. This book is about one woman's thoughts about her mind, body, and soul.

This book openly shares this woman's issues related to her marriage, health, sickness, and spiritual development. It's about darkness, strongholds, spiritual warfare, grief, loss, anger, resentment and rage. The book describes this woman's experiences with parenting, marital, and occupational stressors. In addition, it will be sharing the ways that this woman coped with living in a fast paced and ever changing society.

The purpose of this book is to help others who have faced similar challenges. It is written as a testimony and to provide, motivation, inspiration and encouragement. Sunnie admits that she met with opposition as she prepared to write this book. Family and friends advised her that she would be taking a risk exposing her life in this way. However, Sunnie felt compelled to tell her story.

The struggles Sunnie Davis had trying to make sense of the pressures and forces from within and outside forces have almost levelled her to the ground. Her eighty-two year old mother always told her, "Just because you fall down, doesn't mean you have to stay down there.... just get back up and dust yourself off and keep it moving." As Sunnie states "my mother is such a wise, intelligent and beautiful woman and it's her strength, tenacity and encouragement which have kept me going for all these many years." Sunnie loves her mother so dearly.

In fact about one year ago, Sunnie was praying to God, "Lord you know that mama is getting older and she is my best friend, and I am closer to her than anyone else on this earth…what's going to happen to me once she is gone?" She further went on to say, "God I could not bear that loss... you have to make me stronger to deal with losing her as I could not bear that loss."

Sunnie learned to be careful what she asked for. In this case, she got a challenge which would test her faith and change the course of her life from that point on. Shortly thereafter is when her life took a turn for the worse and she believed that she would die due to the physical and mental issues she developed. However, before going any further, I must paint a picture of exactly who Sunnie Davis is and the many trials and tribulations that led her on an ever-changing journey.

As a young woman, Sunnie's mother told her that she had only planned on having three children. Sunnie sees herself as a miracle baby. Altogether Sunnie's mother had 7 children. Back in those days, birth control was not readily available. Her mother did not believe in abortions. While her mother was pregnant with Sunnie she got saved and filled with the Holy Ghost. At conception Sunnie believes she had God's mercy and grace.

Sunnie is the middle child of seven children. She has two older sisters and four brothers, (two younger and two older). Growing up they were a very close- knit family. Sunnie loved her siblings and her parents in spite of her many challenges and struggles growing up in the sixties and early seventies. God has shown Sunnie's family favour and today as she writes this book, everyone in her family is still alive, "praise the Lord."

Sunnie's immediate family/siblings are very private and would probably prefer that she not mention their names in this book. They would prefer that she not discuss the details of their upbringing and the not so pleasant aspects of their lives.

Sunnie indicates that part of her wants to respect their wishes. The other part of her feels like she needs to be honest based on her own perceptions, experiences and childhood memories. This book is written to help others who may have faced the same or similar challenges. To let them know that they are not alone in their struggle. **For the remainder of this book it will be Sunnie's voice telling her story.**

"Another thing my mama taught me a long time ago was, you just can't go around trying to please everybody so you might as well please yourself." "Make yourself happy."

What she said is true, but somehow I have never internalized these words. My illnesses (mental and physical) have caused me a great deal of pain. Trying to present an image to the world as a little girl until a woman that I had it all together, but as a child I felt alone, misunderstood, abandoned and rejected.

CHAPTER 2

"TRY HARD TO GET ALONG"

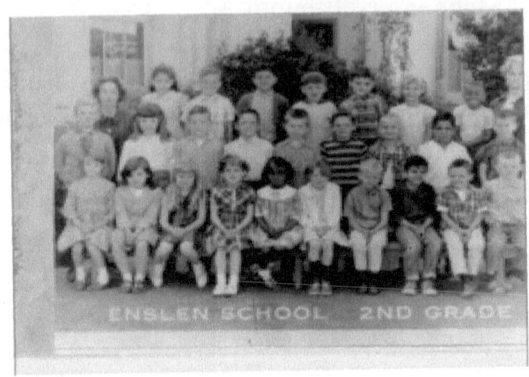

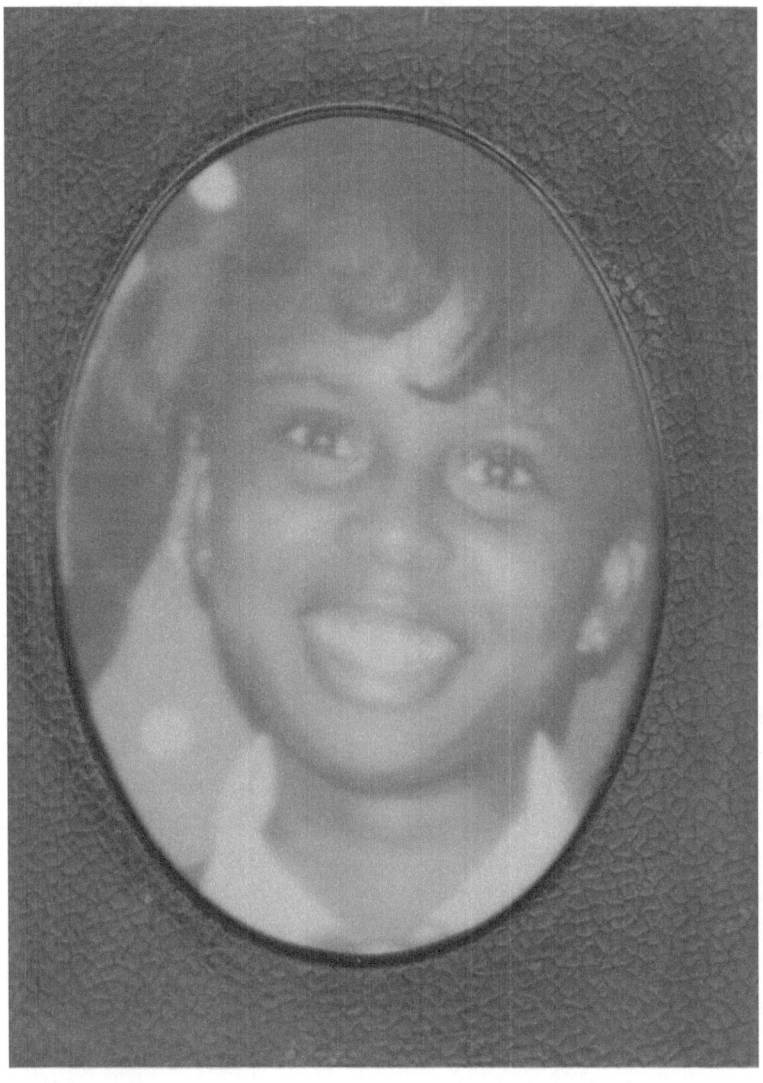

During the height of the civil rights movement, I was seven years old. We moved from Bakersfield, CA to Modesto, CA in 1966. The neighbourhood that we moved to was on the west side in Modesto, California. It consisted of a mixture of people: blacks, whites, and Mexicans and a very few Asians. This was a culture shock for me as a little girl. When I was in the first grade in Bakersfield, I attended an all-black school. The teachers were white, but they were supportive and encouraging.

In August of 1966, Sunnie, at age seven had to integrate by way of a bus to an all-white school. The integration laws were just being established. Sarcastically speaking, I was one of the lucky ones." I was the only one in my family that had to go to the predominantly white school. It was more than an hour drive each way to and from school. My six other siblings went to a totally different school in the neighbourhood we lived in. There was only one other black male child who attended the predominantly white school, and he was my neighbor. We were the only two black kids in the entire segregated school. In addition, we made history as we were the first black children to attend the segregated school.

Thinking back on those days, is not pleasant for me as I still remember the fear I had from looking at all those white kids staring me down on the first day of school. Just try to imagine in 1963 just three years prior, south Carolina's Clemson college became the first integrated public school in that state. Governor George C. Wallace of Alabama stood in a doorway at the university of Alabama in a symbolic attempt to block two black students from enrolling in 1963, his attempt failed. Similarly, I felt like those individuals where possibly just as frightened as I was being only seven years old.

It was quite obvious that the white kids did not want me on their bus. They also did not want me at their school. Their parents probably fed them a bunch of nonsense about black people and they did not want me or the other black child at their school.

My teacher who was also white made it very clear to me that she did not like me and the only reason I was at that school was because it was the law.

What does that do for a little girl's psyche, mind, soul and spirit at seven years old? My ignorant teacher did not want to touch me, nor my hand to show me how to hold a pencil to write my ABC's; so guess what? I had to teach myself. My penmanship was terrible then and it still is to this day.

I remember thinking that my teacher looked like a mean witch from "The Wizard of Oz" movie. I was afraid of her. When I raised my hand to ask a question, she did not respond. She instead looked over my head to the next student. When it was time to feed the classroom's pet turtle, the teacher asked for volunteers, I raised my hand; but again the teacher never picked me to feed the pet turtle.

Little by little, I was losing what little self-esteem I had developed in the first six years of my life. I developed a social-phobia, school phobia, anxiety and depression.
From those early experiences, I can still visualize one of my peers; she had long brown hair and every day after school she threatened to "kick my butt". She called me the "n-word", "blackie" and spit at me. Every day she would literally chase me down when I got off the bus to walk home.

Unfortunately due to these overwhelming stressors I was held back that year and had to repeat the second grade the following year. Today God is enlightening me and showing me that my fear, loneliness, anger and rage was being stuffed deep down inside at that early age and I continued to internalize those emotions for the next fifty years of my life. I truly only wanted to be loved and accepted. I was innocent and a child should not have to deal with the harshness of racism at such an early age.

In spite of those negative experiences, God was in the midst of it all. He told me not to worry. He sent the comforter when I was so lonely, afraid and anxious. He sent the comforter in the way of two little white boys who would walk with me, and would protect me from those other children. I remember one of the nice kids gave me a ride on his bicycle to avoid the bullying.

Some may wonder why my mother or father didn't intervene on my behalf. You have to remember, black folks did not have many rights at that time.

This was the early sixties and many blacks saw integration as a positive thing to produce equality of the races. After all, Martin Luther King Jr. gave many speeches about integration and my parents admired dr. king and his messages.

They saw this as progression instead of oppression. They were saddened by the assassination of Dr. Martin Luther king Jr. and John F. Kennedy.

I remember the day Dr. King was killed as we watched it on TV. We were all speechless and numb. I'll never forget the look on my father's face. My mother also looked so sad and was overwhelmed with grief and sadness. My mother said to look to the cross for peace.

My mother use to tell me: "Sunnie, just try hard to get along." that's when I learned to start faking it, going out of my way to make friends, smiling instead of crying when what I was feeling was anger, sadness, and rage. Rejection, fear and loneliness had taken root in my soul. I learned how to make a few friends by being super nice and funny. But that was little comfort for the constant bullying. Eventually my mother did go to the school after I started crying and saying, I don't want to go to school."

She talked to the principal and the principal allowed me to start going to the elementary school in my neighborhood which was very diverse. I quickly became popular and was accepted by the white students as well as the other races. By the way, one may ask, "why didn't your father speak up for you?" In my opinion in the sixties the black man was seen more as a threat than the black woman and so my mother handled all the school matters related to their children.

Besides my father was working ten to twelve hours per day to ensure we had food on our table and paying the mortgage, and all the other house hold bills. One might say he was a workaholic. My family, like other families, had skeletons in the closet that we just did not talk about. My mother as I have already stated was a Godly woman who was in church most of the time. My father on the other hand, drank too much (he was an alcoholic), was in my opinion physically abusive, a harsh disciplinarian, hung out with his friends, and gambled. He was present physically but absent emotionally.

When he came home from work, I learned to read his moods by observing his facial gestures and ques. In my opinion, he really did not know how to parent me and my siblings as we needed to be parented due to his alcoholism. He could not teach me how to love as his parents probably were unable to demonstrate love outwardly towards him. The curse had been passed down from one generation to the next. Now some may argue that my father showed his love by being a great provider. Being a provider is one thing, but for a child who was very sensitive, I wanted and needed more.

As a child, I needed to feel love by my parents showing me affection, emotional attentiveness, and nurturing. Today I describe that as my "love language." my family was not perfect, but today I don't hold any anger or resentment toward my parents. They did the best they could with their own past life experiences, family dynamics, psychological, social/cultural knowledge and education. As an adult, I later learned that my father had a similar upbringing in which his father used to whip him and his siblings and by today's standards child protection laws he too would have been considered as physically abusive.

I remember my dad told me that his father had a son from a previous marriage and his brother's mother passed away. Afterwards, my grandfather married father's mother. His older half-brother was about 10 years old and my dad was about 7. My father said that his half-brother was very jealous of my dad and was angry that he had lost his biological mother. My dad said "my brother use to tell lies on me all the time to get me into trouble. Unfortunately, my grandfather could not see my uncle's deceptive ways and as a result, he would severely beat my dad to "teach him a lesson".

At eighty-five years old, my father's voice cracked as he re-called those events. It made me want to cry for him. In talking to my dad now, I am not afraid of him anymore. He is such a different person than who I remembered as a child. He is so humble, meek and mild mannered now. He does not raise his voice and he tells me every time that I talk with him that he loves me. He says I love you and I love all of my children." this makes me want to cry as I type these words as I longed to hear those words as a child. I just never felt loved by my father as girl.

The relationship between a daughter and her father is so special because it impacts the child's self-esteem and worth. Without that perceived love and support, the female child will likely seek that love from a male as she becomes a young woman into adulthood. At times I questioned my mother if I had been adopted. She would laugh and tell me "you know you look too much like your brothers and sisters to be adopted." as a matter of fact most people said I looked just like my dad.

In terms of the whippings, that was passed down from one generation to the next. I personally believe that black people whipped their kids as they modeled their slave masters who beat their slaves. My ancestors only perpetuated what was done to them. I know that this is a controversial subject; however, with the thousands of cases of child abuse reported each year, an alternative to whippings is worth considering. I swore I would never beat my child as I did not want my child to grow up in fear as I did, and I wanted her to love me.

It was also difficult for me at home being the middle child. I often felt ignored and neglected from my siblings, especially my older siblings. They did not want me hanging around them, and I was teased constantly and called silly nicknames like "moonshine and forehead." They said I had a large forehead. Today I see it as a symbol of beauty. Back then I always wore bangs to cover my fore head. Looking back at those home experiences, my family loved to tease each other not just me. But back then with the issues I had at the school, and then at home, only intensified my feelings of insecurity and shame.

As a child growing up, I can remember my first panic attack. I was walking on the sidewalk and my neighbor who was much older than I was walking with some of his friends. They began to tease me as they had seen my siblings do that to me so frequently. My heart started beating really fast and I experienced intense fear like I would have a heart attack. I would have many similar experiences happen like that throughout my childhood and later as an adult.

People always thought I was so happy. I learned early on how to be the class clown. I had a big smile and decent looking white teeth. At my integrated school I made friends easily. I began to make jokes and pretend like I was always happy. I began to be told that I was humorous by my friends and cute. This helped my self-esteem and I soon learned that people liked me for my personality. I then began to use charm and talent for acting to gain popularity and it worked.

My grades were now good and my teachers liked me. It's amazing how my self- worth improved when I learned how to make others like me. To be honest, I actually began to love school as I became very social. I got involved in choir, orchestra (I played the violin) and cheerleading.

I moved into the white kids' circles as well as the black kids' circles. I mastered the art of doing that without being called an "Oreo" by the black kids. Some of my friends were not so lucky. Some of my black friends went too far trying to be accepted by their white peers at the risk of alienating themselves from their black peers. There is a fine line to master that art and I somehow did it with ease.

I can recall in high school when I tried out to be a cheerleader. It was something that I really wanted; I realized that it was based on popularity more than talent. I had tried out previously and lost. So I made friends with a very popular white girl who had been a cheerleader for years. She adored me. She took me under her wings and taught me everything she knew about cheerleading. She then introduced me to all her friends and all of a sudden, I was super popular. I still had to prove myself and had to demonstrate skills and talent.

I auditioned for cheerleader and the student body voted for me. I often heard it said you need talent for when opportunity knocks on your door. The late James Brown said it best by his song lyrics: I don't want anybody to give me nothing, open up the door, and I'll get it myself." Some would call it manipulative; however, I learned at an early age how to play the game as others have done it for centuries. It was called "the good ol' boy network" or "it is not what you know, but who you know" when I was growing up, I use to hear others say "you have to know somebody to get a job for that company... you just can't have the degrees, skills and talents; if you don't know somebody, you will not get a job for that company."

Politics is not something that I enjoy, but I understand that it is the way of the world that we live in and I am just trying to survive like the next person.

Today I don't want to harbor any negative feelings about those early child hood memories. The Lord is still working with me on my anxiety, anger, and rage. I realize that it is necessary to forgive if I want to be healthy.

CHAPTER 3

MY YEARS AS AN ACTOR

The most eventful thing which changed my life forever was when Ms. Jones, a black school counselor, began the first Miss Black Teenager of Modesto pageant in 1977. I was seventeen years old and she encouraged me to participate in the pageant. I did and I took home the title of "Miss Black Teenager of Modesto," I won the talent competition for writing and developing my own interpretation of the character "Kizzy" from Alex Haley's book "roots."

I was voted "miss congeniality" by my peers and won the "spirit" award by the pageant committee. From that experience, I went on to compete in the Miss Black Teenager World pageant in Roanoke, VA. I was one of the finalists. I flew alone on an airplane for the first time at age seventeen and saw a whole new world. I saw other young ladies who were also young, gifted, talented and black.

I saw black businesses owners and entrepreneurs, doctors, and attorneys. This was a whole new world for me and it helped me to develop self-esteem and self-worth beyond my wildest imagination. I was now on my way.

Many years later after graduating from high school, I would repeatedly audition for parts and would usually get picked as lead actors in plays. I can recall being asked by the head of the cultural and arts department to play the role of Winnie Mandela.

I gladly accepted the offer and I performed in the black theatre and talent show case at California State University Fresno. It was very powerful as I was able to give my interpretation of Winnie Mandela while she was still married to Nelson Mandela.

This was positive as it showed the love between the two of them while he was yet in prison. This was a love story. Since it was a monologue, I had to remember long lines as I was the only person talking throughout the presentation. There were several other monologues, singing, and poetry readings. I say this humbly but my acting stood out as I won the best actor award for my performance. I still have the trophy and it's a reminder to me that I was a good actor.

In 1988, I auditioned to perform in "The Wiz" the black rendition of The Wizard of Oz. This was a Broadway musical which was initially opened in New York. However, the play was at "Roger Rocha's musical hall in Fresno. I was selected to portray the good witch "Addaperle." Two of my co-actors have won tony awards and are starring in block buster movies. I am truly happy for them; but once again, there are times when I say, I wonder what it would be like if I had not been too afraid to move to the places where movies are made." It's never too late some stars don't become famous until their middle age or older. We will see.

In 1992 I portrayed the character Ruth in "A Raisin in the Sun" I loved that character. Her lines were rich with emotions, laughter sadness, loss and grief, and rage. We performed in a large local theater and my family came from Modesto to see me in that play.

I received accolades for my performance which made me want to pursue my acting career; I would love to hear people tell me that I was so believable as the character I portrayed; or that my performance was riveting. It made me long to do acting on the big screen. However, for some reason, I never felt God's leading to pursue an acting career.

At least not to pack my bags to move to Hollywood or New York. Sometimes we don't understand God's plan. I know that the desire was there, and God opened doors for me to act in my local community. Perhaps he did not want me to move to Hollywood or New York as he knew my personality.

It is possible that I would not survive in those environments. I often think about that movie "The Preacher's Daughter"; for those unfamiliar with the movie it was basically about a young woman who moved away from her small town in hopes to become an actor/singer. She left the church upbringing to end up using drugs and alcohol and found herself in an abusive relationship.

When I saw some of my peer actors on television that I performed with in those earlier years, I used to feel some envy. I performed with actors who moved to Hollywood or New York and are in major motion movies today; others have gone to New York Julliard's School of Performing Arts and have won Tony Awards. Most of these people are younger than I am. God has shown me that I probably would not have survived Hollywood.
He has shown me that my personality is very sensitive and that I may not have been able to handle the rejection that actors often have to face. He has also shown me that I get depressed easily.

As an actress, one must be very confident and willing to have several doors slammed in their faces. When I think of those things, I tell myself it probably was not for me to become an actress in Los Angeles or New York. Fame is not for everyone. I hate to rationalize or make excuses for not pursuing my God given talent. Today I just ask the Lord if it's your will for me to act, I pray that it is in commercials so that I will be able to earn an income.

Community Theater is fun, but it is quite exhausting doing the same show over and over again without pay. I am not a "spring chick" anymore and I think the commercials would be less time consuming while earning an income. Lord let your will be done in my life and may I not be blinded related to my true God given talent and what I am supposed to do with it.

In 1992, I was given the opportunity to travel with the California State University, Fresno Acting Troop to Africa. I was cast to play several characters in "El Hajj Malik" others may know his other name Malcolm X. The acting troop traveled to Africa.

It was a great experience for me. It was powerful when I got off the airplane and I saw the big ocean which possibly transported my ancestors to America. I got goose bumps as I looked at the many Nigerians who spoke in their native tongues and I wondered what it would be like to be able to speak in my ancestors' native tongues. Another thing I loved was the food, music and the cultural arts and crafts that the people created to sell in the markets.

To see young children working at such a young age also was very enlightening for me. In the USA, young children were not allowed to work without work permits; however, these young children were being taught at an early age about entrepreneurship. Not to mention, this was what was expected in order to survive.

In 1996, I was asked to play one of the sisters in the stage play "Having Our Say" a two-person cast which was a wonderful story about two black women who were sisters who lived beyond 100 years old. One sister was a dentist and the other was a teacher. I played the role of the teacher. My friends and family traveled from my home town to Fresno to see me. This really made me feel special. From that point on, I was in several commercials, radio advertisements and public service announcements while living in Fresno, California.

CHAPTER 4

GROWING UP IN THE CHURCH

Born and raised in the church, I learned to express myself musically and with an instrument. I saved up blue chip stamps (some of you are too young to know what I am talking about.) When mama purchased something at the grocery store, she was given a blue- chip stamp book to fill with the stamps.

Once the book was filled, we could buy goods from a catalogue. I saved the blue-chip stamp book and bought my first tambourine. I loved playing my tambourine in church.

It was fun and it helped me to stay awake. We belonged to a church of God In Christ (Pentecostal) church. My mother was a Sunday school teacher, secretary, youth leader, and she basically held every position there was to hold at our church.

We joined that church in 1966 and to this day, my mother attends that same church; approximately fifty years later. She never bounced around from one church to another. She always said "there is not a perfect church out there. You have to take the good with the bad." She now holds the title of "Mother Davis." She is a prayer warrior and is sought after by her church members for spiritual guidance and leadership.

My mother is my best friend. She loves me in spite of any flaws I carry today. She has taught me to be leery and careful of whom you pick as your friends. Mama also said, "You can't put all your trust and faith in your pastor. Check out what he/or she is saying by reading the bible for yourself, and if what the pastor is saying is not of God, you will know and follow what God teaches us." I have learned that I can't put all my trust in man, as he may disappoint me each and every time.

I also sang in the church choir which sometimes only consisted of three to four people. We did not have a band or an orchestra. The most we had then were tambourines, drums, organ and a piano. In addition, our church congregation was small about thirty to forty people at most.

You see, we come from a small community where everybody knew each other's' business. By this time, all of my older brothers and sisters had graduated from high school and had moved away and no longer attended our church. So it was just me, and my two younger brothers. We had to attend Sunday school and stay in church for long hours from 9:30am to 3:30pm or later at times.

The church members sold   dinners to raise money for the church. We attended choir practice on the weekends and youth group during the week. When mama went to church, the three youngest siblings were right there. Our nick names at that time were the "three little ones." I remember one time saying to myself, I can't wait to turn eighteen, so that I can stop going to church… as I will be grown and I won't have to live at home and go to church." Growing up in our home, we ate the best meat as my father was a butcher. He brought home mostly beef and pork from his packing house. My father knew how to cook really well as did my mother. I use to watch my father cook fried fish, stews, and barbeque.

 He would also broil steak, smoke fish, turkey and a variety of meats. My father was also a hunter so he would hunt for venison, fowl, and rabbit, etc. My father took care of his family again by providing for us. My father and mother both were from the south so they could cook such a variety of food that we loved food and all the celebrations in our home involved my parents cooking something special.

As I came home from school, I can fondly remember at thanksgiving, my mother cooking homemade dressing. I could smell the onions, bell pepper, and celery she sautéed these ingredients to make the dressing. The aroma filled our house and I could even smell the food from outside. She allowed me to help her by chopping up the vegetables to put in the cornbread mixture.

My favorite was the dressing with giblet/liver gravy. My mother knew how to make liver taste good. For New Year's we would have gumbo and or chit'lins or chitterlings if you want to say it another way (smile). When I was a kid, I did not like greens, other vegetables; however, today I love soul food, and I have been told by my husband that I am an excellent cook.

My siblings including my brothers all know how to cook very well. This is something that my family takes great pride in: our ability to cook good food. This trait has been passed down through the generations. My father's mother was a great cook and often baked cakes from scratch (not store bought). One of my father's brothers owns a soul food restaurant and my brother's daughter is studying to become a chef.

CHAPTER 5

KNOW THYSELF: NEVER TRY TO
WALK IN ANOTHER'S
FOOTSTEPS

As I am writing this book right now, I am praying for the Holy Spirit intervention to guide my words as I share them with you. Guide and lead me as I speak from my heart the unadulterated truth on behalf of Jesus my Lord and saviour, my family, and my friends and colleagues. As a little girl, I always knew I had a special calling to do something great. I have always sensed it would be something related to the creative arts, music, entertainment and a little voice (the Holy Spirit) has always told me I would someday write a book. Yes, this is the truth.

I have kept a journal since I was in the sixth grade and throughout my life especially during times of stress, confusion, anxiety, depression, brokenness, and relationship issues... I have also loved photography and have pictures of myself, my family from as far back as I can remember. Every time I took pictures, I would jokingly say, "This picture may be put in my book that I am going to write." I also knew that I would be speaking on a stage either acting or motivating others.

Interestingly enough, Satan has always tried to tell me that I was not smart enough to write a book. This stems from my early days in elementary school being held back a grade. Being held back really bothered me which made me feel inadequate. I am always trying to prove myself to others and have a tendency to want to be perfect.

Although I have kept journals, this is the first time I have decided to put some of my journal writing into a book form. I must say that it has been quite a journey. I have avoided and procrastinated about why I could not write this book. The devil does not want me to be successful. I know that but for me it's "sink or swim "and at this time, I am swimming like a fish.

My book title is simply: "My Journey." God knows what's best and he is still the author of what is to take place in my life and on his schedule, not my schedule. This is my journey not anyone else's so I just need to remember that as I write this book. If God is for us, who can be against us? Thank you Jesus!!!!

From elementary to intermediate school, I tried to follow in my two older sisters' footsteps by taking business related classes. Back in the early sixties and seventies, young black girls were encouraged to take typing, home economic and shorthand. Basically we were encouraged to take secretarial courses.

At age fourteen I got my work permit and got a job through a grant funded program called summer youth employment program. It was designed for youth from low income families. The purpose of the program was to also teach young underserved youth job skills and career development. We met the criteria. My mother was a stay at home mom, (homemaker) and there were nine of us including my parents.

My first job was a custodian assistant. All the office jobs were already taken by my peers. I did not want to do that work at the time. However, I saw a yellow ten speed bike that I wanted, and the only way I was going to get that bike was to pay for it by working. I did not like to get my hands dirty, I was feminine back then and I continue to be today. Ironically, I like gardening now so I have gotten over getting my hands dirty. God is good. I bought my yellow ten speed bike. I only had to work as a custodian for about two weeks. Then I was moved into an office clerk position. While going to high school, I held these jobs: librarian assistant, telephone operator for my high school and office assistant.

As a senior, I got a job as a sales associate for Macy's department store. By this time I was driving and had saved enough money to purchase my own car. It was yellow and very sporty. So I had a yellow ten speed bike and now a yellow car. It was a Capri but those cars are not made anymore.

CHAPTER 6

FINDING MY PLACE UNDER THE SUN

By the time I got into high school, my oldest sister decided she would major in Business Administration. I looked up to her and thought she was so smart I wanted to be like her. I think it also stems from my low self-worth back then. I also wanted to play it safe and not veer off too much from what she was doing. My other sister was also very smart. She majored in Public Administration and worked in a bank.

She later got her BA in Public Administration. I guess you could say that I wanted to be accepted and admired as I saw the community and my parents admire and speak highly of my sisters. As a result, when it was time for me to go to college, I tried to major in business. In 1978 to 1980 I went to Modesto Junior College. I registered for the business administration course track. To be honest, I hated those classes. Math, accounting, economics, statistics and anything related to business, I hated it. Trying to emulate my older sisters caused me much distress. I was getting poor grades in those courses; I just could not grasp the concepts. I was out of my comfort zone and I knew it.

The only course that I liked out of all the courses was typing. I learned how to use the keyboard without looking at my fingers and I was a very fast typist and having typing skills, enabled me to get jobs throughout my career. Employers generally sought after individuals with typing speed and accuracy.

In 1980, I was about twenty-one and that is when I decided to change my major from business to social science. I actually went to see the career counselor and she gave me a vocational assessment to determine my career aptitude skills.

She advised me that I would do well in courses/careers related to counseling, motivational speaking, teaching, helping others succeed and reach their full potential. It was based on that evaluation, that I changed my major to social science. The school counselor also suggested that I see the college psychiatrist as she noticed that I was anxious and I told her that I had bouts of depression.

The psychiatrist, Dr. Brown, prescribed me Inderral for anxiety and I kept that a secret from my family and friends due to the stigmatization of taking medications for depression and or anxiety.

All I needed was to get someone else's view about how they saw my strengths and potential. I decided to change my major to psychology, and social work. I excelled in those, I was comfortable and I felt that I was in my zone. I liked these courses because I was trying to heal from my childhood experiences of feeling rejected and abandoned. Social work dealt with biological, psychological, social, spiritual, cultural and environmental systems courses.

CHAPTER 7

PRINCESSES HAD TO KISS SOME FROGS

I had a fantasy about love. I only had two boyfriends in high school. I did not start to blossom as a pretty girl until after high school. I was considered cute, but the boys that I liked did not appear interested in me. There were boys that liked me. They were nice enough but I did not feel that sparkle, and magnetism towards them that I had seen in love stories on TV.

The guys I wanted to talk to (go out with) did not appear interested in me. I was considered a "good girl" or a goody two shoe and the entire community I lived in knew my family. Not to mention that I had four brothers who were protective of their sister. But as a junior in high school I wanted to go to the Turkey Trot (similar to the prom). I did not have a boyfriend and I needed one to go to that dance. There was not much interracial dating in high school and the black guys my age were either nerds, or bad boy types. That did not leave me with many options. I ended up dating a guy just to go to the Turkey Trot and then broke up with him after that as we really did not have much in common. He seemed nice enough but there were no sparks for me.

He appeared to like me more than I liked him and the boys that I was really attracted to would be the bad boy type. This became a pattern for me. Again not having a close relationship with my father as a young woman impacted my self-esteem. This appeared to continue to haunt me throughout my dating years. As a senior, my second boyfriend was not attractive to me, but again, I wanted a boyfriend so I dated him just to say I had a boyfriend. Believe it or not, he was a minister. He was only a couple of years older than I was. He was more advanced than I was. I was a virgin and he tried his hardest to change that, but I had no intentions of getting pregnant. My plan was to be successful and attend college, and after I graduated from college, I planned on getting married and having children. I eventually broke up with him after a couple of months.

After high school, I started attending a non-denominational church (we believed in the father and the son, and the Holy Spirit but it was not as strict as the Pentecostal church that I was raised. I was going to church and was a Christian. However, the church I was going to was very small and I was being taught the word; but still did not have a boyfriend. Again, it was important for me to have a boyfriend. I know now that those thoughts stemmed from low self-worth and my need for love and approval from my father who did not outwardly demonstrate he loved me from an emotional stance; however he did from a provider's perspective. Unfortunately, this lack of outwardly demonstration of love and affection caused me to turn for approval from males.

My self-esteem was always tied to being loved or liked by a male and I always felt incomplete without a boyfriend. At my church, I saw my friends hooking up with guys and dating. I thought to myself, "This is getting old"; I want to be in a relationship too. Initially I was "on fire" for God. That was slang for really believing in the word and spreading God's message of love, peace, mercy and grace. I even recruited several of my college friends to come to church with me.

Unfortunately, I began to become discouraged and somewhat disillusioned while attending my church. My pastor taught about being "unevenly yoked" or put another way Christians dating or marrying others who were not Christians. I saw my college buddy's dating whomever they wanted to and doing whatever they wanted to in their relationships. Here I was trying to be the good Christian young woman; however, when I saw my college/Christian friends dating, I became bitter and somewhat envious. I decided to call some of my old friends from high school and suggested that we go to a night club. In my mind I knew that it was wrong as a Christian young woman to go to the club and to start behaving the way I did when I was not saved. But at this point, I was tempted by the devil to back slide and that's just what happened.

I met a guy in the club that was not in the church. He said he believed in God but he was not living a Godly life. I thought he was fine. He was bi-racial (black and white) and he was charming, about six feet tall and was very sexy to me. We began to date and he asked me to be his girlfriend. One thing led to another, and I stopped going to church as I felt I had betrayed God. I did not want to be a hypocrite, so I just stopped going altogether. I also could not bear the fact of the disappointing God for my un-Godly lifestyle.

After earning my BA and completing college 1982, Ronald Reagan got into office and the entire grant funded programs for people of color were extinguished. Social service types of jobs were not available as they were before the Reagan administration. The jobs had dried up and I found myself with a degree, but unable to get a job. The only jobs that were available for people with degrees in social science were history teachers or those with early elementary school teaching credentials. I wanted to be a counselor; but was advised the best way to make that happen was to get a teaching credential. I decided to go back to school to get a teaching credential. I was accepted in the teaching credential program at California State University, Stanilaus in 1982.

In the teaching program you had to take curriculum courses as well a student teach (going into the classroom and learning how to teach from your master teacher) and I substituted as a teacher with a BA degree, and I found that I really did not like the confinement of a classroom. I felt like I had made a terrible career move again. I was still living near the campus in an apartment by myself in Turlock, CA directly across the street from California State University of Stanislaus. I was still in the teaching program when the university had a huge job fair where there were recruiters from various large companies in the central California area. I decided to go to the career /job fair to see what was available. Little did I know that my life was about to make a very big shift.

I was recruited by a black district manager to work for a large department store in Fresno, California. The pay was excellent and I needed a job at this point. I did not like the teaching program so I had to make a decision quickly as the recruiter was only there for two days. I decided to jump for the opportunity.

I had had some retail experience working for Macy's while in high school. The district manager made it seem so great. He described the benefits and the promise that I would be trained as a manager. The company basically paid for my move and I moved to Fresno, California. I was alone and started pursuing a career as a department store assistant manager. I was basically a glamorized sales associate. Wow!!! It was not a good idea to accept that job I thought, "Here I am again doing business type of work which was not good for me." Numbers and I were not a good match and as a store manager, I had to know how to do the numbers. One of the good things about being recruited was that it got me out of Turlock, CA.

On a positive note, I move to Fresno, CA. Which had a lot more to offer academically as California State University, Fresno was there, and there were multiple churches to choose from; although I had stopped going to church out of guilt and shame. God has a way of turning our mistakes into something positive or he has mercy on us. Fresno was like a big city to me compared to Modesto; it was a metropolitan city with cultural diversity, community and social activities, jazz concerts, R&B concerts, a major university and the job market was also better there.

I can't leave out the fact that there were a whole lot of guys, and I was going to the clubs every weekend; hanging out with my co-workers that I had met on my job doing all the things that I was taught was wrong as a Christian woman. Oh yeah, and that boyfriend that I had met in Turlock, I became disinterested in him when I met another guy who I thought had more potential than my boyfriend from Turlock, CA. Again, I thought this new guy was fine; he had an Audi 5000 and he use to let me drive it. I became very materialistic. I started to like men who I thought had money, and material possessions.

I dated this man for about six months and then he started treating me very badly. When we first met, he wined and dined me but after six months he stopped calling me when he said he would. He started avoiding me, and said that I was too clingy. He even went behind my back and told one of my friends that I was too needy so he decided to break up with me. I guess it is true "you reap what you sow" Another way of looking at this is "what goes around comes around."

I was devastated. I thought I was in love but actually I was in lust. I had made a deal with the devil and sold my soul to him. I paid dearly for disobeying God. I had multiple relationships after that and they all had the same feel to me. The guys would start out very charming, wining and dining me, buying me flowers, nice gifts and jewelry. Everything would be going great, and then they would do a disappearing act. The phone calls would stop, the gifts would stop, and once again I would feel disillusioned, abandoned, and rejected. I had the nice apartment, a nice car, and a good job; but would always have men problems.

In looking back at my journey, I appeared to pick the same type of men as my father; at times my father was cold, aloof, and non-expressive. The times that I saw him laugh and joke were when he had been drinking. The men I liked had good jobs, but they were womanizers. They made promises that they could not keep.

By this time, I had been working for another company in retail management. I had become very shapely, cute, smart and feisty; initially, the men I dated seem to like me but for the wrong reasons. Looking back, the men appeared to like me physically, but were not into me emotionally. The relationships would start out with the electricity, passion, and sparks that I had seen in the movies; unfortunately, the sparks would die out after about six months. My Christian life was put on the back burner as I was living a conflictual lifestyle. I knew that God would not condone my lifestyle and behaviors.

I knew that my life was not in the will of God. I had several unsuccessful relationships where the men used me for one thing and then broke up with me or just stopped calling. It seemed that all the men who wanted to talk to me were cheaters, married, drug abusers, or nerds. On the outside looking in from my family's perspective, friends, and co-workers, I had a perfect life. I had the degrees, nice apartment, car, nice clothes/jewelry, and a good job. But my love life sucked.

I was independent. However, I never felt complete. I know now that the completeness that I was looking for could only be filled by God. Unfortunately, for several years I kept looking outside of myself and for men to fill that void.

There was one relationship that really messed me up emotionally. I had fallen deeply in love with a man I met while working in the retail management job. His name was Ricky. He was dark chocolate with big dreamy eyes and kept his hair nicely groomed. I thought he was the finest man I had ever seen and I believed that it was love at first sight. I thought the feeling was mutual. He also worked for the same retail store where I was employed; our relationship became a whirl wind and he swept me off of my feet. I allowed him to move in with me and my roommate. That was one of the biggest mistakes I made. In all my years of dating, I swore I would never "shack up" with anyone." I was not raised that way. They say that love is blind and in this case I was so blind. This man used me like no other. He stole my TV and bought drugs. One night after work I came home, and my front door was wide opened. I can recall slowly walking up the stairs as I lived on the second floor of two story apartments. I feared that maybe a home intruder was still there. My heart was beating rapidly as I approached the front door. I walked in and saw that my TV was gone. I sat in the middle of the floor and cried. I knew that it was not an intruder. Who was I kidding? I knew that it was my "boyfriend". One time; this same boyfriend took my car and was gone for three days and I had to catch the bus to work. Another time he stole my rent money from the ATM machine. Ugh!!! What a toxic relationship.

I was at an all-time low in that relationship. I remember an experience which shook me up so much that I actually had a nightmare of an evil spirit (the devil) one night while I lay sleeping and I woke up in a cold sweat screaming and I looked over at my boyfriend and he had the same face of the evil spirit I had just dreamt about. My so-called boyfriend took away all of my dignity, my self-respect, and my self-worth all within about three months' time.

Everyone told me he was no good for me, but I didn't believe it. To make matters worse after falling in love with him, he told me he was married but separated. He played the role of the victim as he told me his wife had left him and moved away and they had three children together. I felt so betrayed; I finally broke off the relationship with this man as my heart could not take all that drama anymore. He came in and out of my life several years after he moved out. It was like he had a spell on me or something. I continued to work for the retail company for about five years and decided I had enough in working in a dead end job.

I eventually went back to college and earned my Master's degree in clinical social work. After all the painful relationships I had experienced, now I had the education and life experiences to be a great therapist. Shortly after graduating with my Master's degree, I got a job working as a counselor for The Associative Center for therapy. I actually enjoyed my work as I felt like I was making a difference in other lives. God was there all along. I was really good at what I did as my clients told me and they kept coming back so I must have been doing something right.

After working in this job for about 3-4 years, I decided to broaden my experience by accepting a job at a community mental health center in Merced California. It was higher paying position and it offered more clinical experienced. I enjoyed the work but I did not like the commute. It was about an hour away from Fresno, CA. After about one year of the commute, I decided I needed to find a job where I lived. I was actually approached by the CEO of the company as she was looking for a therapist and my name had come up. She actually called me at my job in Merced and asked me to interview with her organization. I did and I was hired on the spot.

Initially, I loved my job and the clients I served. My clients would tell my supervisor that they loved me and that I was really helping them change their lives. I gained so much experience on that job; I traveled to conferences all over the USA, stayed in 5 star hotels, and met so many interesting people who also worked in the field of mental health.

I stayed at that job for five years and that's when the stress of the work became so overwhelming, and unhealthy. The work hours were long and tiring. I went to bed with a pager and I had to work with child protective services, and I would have to go pick up kids and place them in foster care sometimes at three a.m. in the morning. I started hating my work. The kids were getting sicker and sicker and many of them had committed severe crimes and I started to fear my own safety as a therapist. The girls would curse at me and call me a "bitch." Their lives were so broken and their families were so dysfunctional and all day long I would have to put out fires.

I was getting older and wanted to settle down, but it seemed like I kept picking the same kind of guys. I liked the good looking men, charming, intelligent and great jobs/careers, but they obviously thought they were prettier than I was. They all seem to be cheaters.

Ironically enough, I dated several guys who majored in business and accounting. I guess it is true, opposites attract. But one appeared to be different. He was a very logical; organized and structured, type of thinker, nothing like me. I was free spirited, creative, artsy, and very spontaneous. I never even kept a budget. He strongly believed in having a budget. I ignored our differences because I was in love. He made me feel so special, and I met him at church. I re-dedicated my life to Christ. He was a Christian and we went to church together. I thought this is it. Finally God has sent me my husband. He told me he wanted me to have his baby. This sounds so immature now. But at that time you have to remember, I was longing to be married and to have a baby. I was 40 and longed to be a mother and experience mother hood. I thought if I don't get pregnant soon, I may not ever have that opportunity. I had reached my career goals and I was thrilled that this man had asked me to have his child. I was so happy that he asked me to have his baby.

Before meeting Mike, I began to fear that I would have to be artificially inseminated. Yes I said it. Many other women, not just black women have made that decision. After doing what I thought was "right" putting my career first was the priority initially; however, I was a professional black woman with a degree. I had bought my own home and by many standards a successful black woman; but childless and husbandless. So yes I tried to get pregnant.

By this time, I was already forty-one and as I already mentioned my biological clock was ticking. I knew that he would marry me if I got pregnant. He was a family guy. I began to rationalize my decision to get pregnant unmarried. Shortly thereafter, I got pregnant and at eight months into the pregnancy, we had a big wedding and I was so happy. My family liked Mike and we both came from big families. I thought things were perfect. He had a great job as a professional and so did I. He had his own house and I had my own house. Our future was looking so bright. Our baby was beautiful and we were flying high. His job required that he travel all over the USA.

CHAPTER 8

THE HONEYMOON IS OVER

About three months into our marriage, I noticed that Mike was not being communicative as he had previously been when we were dating. We really did not get a chance to bond as a couple prior to our baby being born. It seemed like the baby was now the priority and I was not the apple of his eye anymore. We continued to love one another and continued to maintain intimacy for quite some time in our marriage However, being married, raising a child, and working outside of the home began to take its toll on me. I was tired after working all day and then coming home taking care of the household chores and caring for our baby and trying to be the perfect wife. I always made sure I cooked dinner, kept the house cleaned, and tried to satisfy Mike as his wife.

I swore that I would never allow myself to get "fat and comfortable" as I heard other's describe it. Trying to play several roles wife, mother, professional and taking care of the household chores became overwhelming to me. I started to get comfortable in my relationship. Before I had my child, I had a very cute shape and maintained a proportionate size for several years. I won't give exact sizes as size is only relative and it is often measured by European standards. I chose not to subject myself to other's standards of beauty. I think that it is unfair and unrealistic for a person to look and act the same prior to marriage and all the responsibilities that went along with that. Now my husband may describe a different scenario about what he saw transpire. However, I always felt like I could not measure up to looking the same and acting the same prior to our marriage. Reality bites and before I knew it, I had become even more depressed now. I had accepted a position for a mental health center in Atlanta and it was quite taxing.

My role as a mother seemed to take the front seat as it was the most demanding role at that time. It's a challenge to feel sexy when you are trying to wear all the hats I was wearing. Mike began to look at me differently. I felt like Mike had a double standard; as he too gained weight and began to lose his hair as he aged; but I did not criticize him for aging. When he began to shut me out, was moody and grumpy all the time, I begged Mike to go to counseling. He refused. He would simply say, "If you would do what I said, we would not be having these problems." Again God told me not to worry, and I am right beside you, look to the cross and fear not.

Mike soon got a promotion which required us to move from California to New Orleans. There was only one problem, I had been working for a company for four years and I only had one more year to become vested and to draw a pension for retirement. So we discussed it and made the decision for Mike to move and me and our child would stay in California.

Mike moved to New Orleans and lived in an extended stay apartment for one year and he would come visit us on the weekends when he could. That really changed our relationship. I started not trusting him as he grew more and more distant from me. He was a good provider. He paid the bills and took care of his family financially, like my father had done. Emotionally I did not feel that he was present. In addition, we had serious communication issues and the distance just made it worse. He would not talk to me and he would not let me in which caused me to feel isolated, abandoned, rejected, angry, resentful. We began to argue all the time.

I felt so depressed and he was unhappy too. We stayed together for our child. I found myself gaining more and more weight. I had low self-esteem as he no longer looked at me with that sparkle in his eye and eating became sedation for me. One year later, our daughter and I joined Mike in New Orleans and we lived in New Orleans for about three years and then Katrina hit New Orleans.

During the entire time we lived in New Orleans, I felt so isolated and alone. I could not find a job as I was considered an outsider. My self-esteem was also tied with me as a professional, now I was just considered as Mike's wife and his profession took a front seat and my professional identity took a back seat. We eventually moved to Atlanta when Mike got a promotion.

Mike's entire family lived in Atlanta. It was great for him and I liked his family, but Mike appeared to care more about spending all of our free time at his family's house. Every Sunday we would go to his mother house for dinner. I just started feeling resentful. I could only see my family maybe one time per year and every week, Mike was able to see his family. Mike and I were in trouble. We were going to church every Sunday but basically living a double life. The more I begged him to go to counseling, the more stubborn he became. He was so private and guarded; he did not believe in disclosing any of his business to anyone outside of his family. I wished he had a male Christian role model who could reinforce to him the importance of being the head of the household. That would include loving his wife as Christ loves the church. I did my best to be a good wife and mother.

We argued about money and finances from the start. I had been independent for so long. At forty-one when we got married, I told him that I wanted to have separate bank accounts. Even though I loved him, I did not trust him as in my prior relationships the men had stolen money from me, lied to me and cheated on me.

So I had issues with trusting him as a man from the start. I had seen my married friends argue about money so I thought that if we had separate accounts, then he would not try to control me on how I should spend my money. That was big mistake. He went along with it, but he was not happy about it. He thought I was just selfish. If I could do it differently, I would not have chosen to have separate accounts because it caused many conflicts.

It was not the Christian way to start a marriage. It was like we were just roommates. Mike also became very controlling. He was like a dictator. He would tell me that I was not keeping the house clean. He would walk around the house and would try to tell me how to decorate my house and would criticize my decorations. I took pride in my ability to decorate the house and all my friends said I should be an interior decorator so I could not understand why he became so critical.

Plus I had kept something a secret from Mike something about my past while we were dating. He found out accidentally just prior to us getting married. He threatened to call off the wedding. I was devastated, pregnant and we had made all the wedding plans, guests had been invited, bridesmaid dresses were made, and my wedding dress had been made.

We got married, but I think that the secret devastated Mike and he did not trust me from the start of our marriage. I think this secret set the tone of our marriage and then everything went downhill from there.

We all have secrets and some we will take to our graves with us. Mike has issues too with his upbringing and family. He is not as transparent as I am, he has skeletons (lots of them), and out of respect for him and very shaky relationship I will not reveal his family issues /secrets. I will say that his family dynamics have not helped our broken marriage. Our problems just seem to grow worse and worse. We were not communicating. Mike had brought up getting a divorce several times. To be honest our marriage had become dead as a door knob.

My friends walked around like their marriages were perfect so I did not have the courage to even share the trials and tribulations I was going through in my marriage. I am not even sure if we will still be married at the end of this book. Our problems seem overwhelming. Our parenting styles were also so different. After we had our child, he was a strong disciplinarian and he said he believed in corporal punishment. I on the other hand, did not believe in whipping our child due to my own whippings I experienced as a child. It made me feel so afraid and anxious. I wanted different for our child.

Mike only spanked our daughter one time, but he set the stage for the rest of her life. It was he whom she obeyed and she did not listen to me. She basically became manipulative and disrespectful to me her mother as I wanted her to love me and not be afraid of me. In looking back, I should have been stronger and a better disciplinarian.

My relationship with my mother as a teen was a little conflictual, but not to the same degree as with my daughter. One thing I did not do was talk back to my mother. Our daughter was growing up fast, she talked back to me. It's embarrassing for me to admit that I lacked parenting skills as I taught parenting to my clients as a social worker. It's different when it's your own child.

She was not afraid of me and I felt like she disrespected me as her mother. After each argument, she would come back to hug me and would always say I love you mom." I saw it as being manipulative; however, perhaps it was just so uncomfortable for me to hear that as when I was growing up my mother did not tell me she loved me. My daughter appeared as frustrated with me as I was with her. Our communication was not good and this caused major issues between my husband and me.

He wanted me to stand up and be the parent and set boundaries and control our daughter; but by this time, I had a laissez-faire attitude about parenting. My physical and emotional health had deteriorated. I had been so sick to point that I felt like I was going to die. My mental health was impacting my physical health and the doctors kept prescribing me more and more medications without any success. I was referred from one specialist to the next, and the doctors were not communicating to each other about my medications. To be honest, I believe that the medications were making me worse.

We now live in Texas after twelve years of marriage soon to be thirteen years, I have been like a pressure cooker and now I am a volcano exploding every chance I get. I am taking it all out on Mike and our daughter. My job too has stressed me out.

I got a job working as a healthcare professional and I won't mention the name of the company but this job has been so stressful. My broken marriage and my relationship with my daughter has caused me to have a nervous breakdown. I have had to be hospitalized on three separate occasions due to panic attacks and feeling like I was going to die. I have overtaken medications as I have been placed on so many. My sleep has been impaired where I haven't slept for days. I finally told my supervisor I needed time off from work, and when I went to the doctor, I was placed on short term disability.

Now I have been on disability for twelve weeks and according to my doctors, I am still not ready to go back to work. Never before have I felt so helpless and out of control. I think that Mike is in denial about my having a mental decompensation (basically a nervous breakdown) I am now crying as I am writing these words out of despair... I am going to stop right now to continue later. My depression is over taking me right now and I feel a panic attack coming upon me.

When I became sick in January 2014, I thought it was a cold or some upper-respiratory infection. After going to my primary care doctor (PCP), she informed me that I had chronic bronchitis. She placed me on prednisone and Albuteral and gave me a breathing treatment. She also gave me antibiotics. None of which seemed to help improve my condition.

I continued to cough and I was still working at that time. It was quite embarrassing and exhausting to have to repeatedly ask to be excused for coughing. My co-workers and the professional colleagues always had sympathy for me and wondered why I was coughing for so long. The more I coughed; the more meds were prescribed to me.

After about six months of this, I was sent to several specialists. I had so many medications and I found it difficult to remember which meds I had taken. Initially my PCP had diagnosed me with Bronchitis and now she said I had irritable bowel syndrome. After several weeks of treatment without results, my PCP informed me that what I had was not a physical condition but a mental condition. I was a mess. My family did not understand what was wrong with me. I was sick all the time or crying all the time. I was diagnosed with major depression and anxiety disorder.

The more meds I took, the more depressed I became. I remember a time when I was taking a bath and I felt so low and so depressed. I was not suicidal, but felt like I could die accidentally due to the medications that I was on and all the negative side effects I was experiencing.

After I got out of the bath tub, I went and got my bible and put it on my stomach. With tears running down my face, I was sobbing profusely; I cried out to the Lord to heal me of all of my afflictions. I begged the Lord to have mercy on me as I felt like the woman with the issue of blood. I asked the Lord for a sign, anything to show that he was listening to me. My hands have shaken for years due to anxiety. The Lord told me to raise my hands in the air and praise him so I did just that and for the first time in a long time, my hands were not shaking. I saw that as a sign from God that he was listening and I began to have faith that he would heal me.

CHAPTER 9

THE BATTLE IS NOT YOURS IT'S
THE LORD'S

While still working, I found myself trying hard not to get into debates with my co-workers. Everyone was getting on my nerves and I began not holding back and being the nice guy. I felt like I did not know how to set boundaries with my co-workers and I felt like I had become a door mat just as when I was a child. I held my tongue for so long until I could not do it anymore. I realized that saying no was ok sometimes so that others would not take advantage of my kindness.

I had some co-workers who were not very honest and would tell lies about me to get me into trouble with my supervisor. I became overwhelmed as I was working long hours and days just to keep up. The work load was so overwhelming that at times, I would burst into tears after upsetting phone calls. I still would not quit. I kept hoping that things would get better. However, they did not. When I did finally tell my supervisor how I was feeling, it may have been too late; I feared that my job was in jeopardy now.

My husband would tell me, "You handle our daughter... You are the mother. You have to do the hard work to get her to respect you."

My marriage had deteriorated and my child rearing practices were poor at best. My entire world was falling apart all around me and I was in trouble. My husband and I were not communicating at all and he would not support me in trying to get my daughter to obey me. There was no structure in our home.

The truth is that from the time my child was very small; I spoiled her and did not discipline her. I was just so happy to have a baby at forty-one, I wanted her to love me and not be afraid of me as I was with my parents. I vowed that I would not whip my child as I was whipped and it made me a very fearful and anxious child.

I went too far the opposite direction and did not discipline her enough. Now that she is twelve years old, she does not have any respect for me as her mother. At least I don't feel she does. She says that she loves and respects me, but my expectations of her are too high. She also states that I want her to do house chores, but her school schedule is too demanding and she needs to complete her homework and that her school work should be her priority.

Again, I think she is trying to be manipulative. When I talk to my friends who have kids the same age, they all have different takes on this issue. Some say to spank, others say to discipline her by taking away her phone, others say it is me with the issues and not her and that I am trying to parent my child and make her be a partner or roommate by having her do chores as my husband does not enjoy doing the house work and is from the old school where the woman or wife manages the house hold chores.

This is crazy making for me. I feel that I need to teach my daughter how to be responsible and doing the dishes, cleaning her room and doing the laundry will start that process.

Her dad has high expectations for her but, sometimes or most of the time; he is traveling so I am both the mother and the father. It's just a big mess. I really tried to alter my parenting styles to better control her; but somehow, we continue to struggle. Many of my friends who have had teenage girls share my experiences and empathize with me on parenting a teen.

One may wonder how could I have a degree in clinical social work and have a dysfunctional family (poor parenting and marital conflicts). The only answer I can come up with it is more difficult when the problems/issues are within your own family. My primary care doctor explained to me that she does surgery on a weekly basis, but when her husband got a cut on his hand, she almost fainted.

I was getting double messages from the church. I was told to obey my husband as he is the head of household. However, he may be a good provider financially but the emotional, nurturing, and empathic husband does not exist. He tells me, I want my cake and eat it too." I think most people do if they are being honest with themselves. Don't get me wrong, Mike does have a lot on his plate and takes care of our businesses, managing rental properties, and oversees the major financial, retirement, and legal matters in our home.

However, I need to be able to communicate with him on an emotional, spiritual, and social basis. I would try to talk with him prior to him going to work and he would say, "Not now, I need to go to work." When he came home from work, I would say "we need to sit down and talk;" his response would be, I just got home from work… I need some time to relax." As a result, we were not communicating and the resentment of him putting it off really started to irritate me. I found myself having to blurt out what I wanted to say and screaming over whatever he was saying. Then he would tell me to leave and that he needed his space. So you see, I was trying to let him be the man of the house, but he was not fulfilling his role as the head of the house.

On a positive note, Mike would go into the pantry and re-organize it to make it more functional and he will also organized the dish pantries, Tupperware, and the seasonings on the shelf, and he also organized the kitchen to make it more functional. Remember, he is the logical thinker, the organizer and some may describe him as anal. I on the hand am not very organized. He always paid the bills and he worked every day. I felt blessed that he was a hard worker and always ensured that they family had what they needed. I just think in our case opposites attract; he saw it as I changed" but in actually, I did not change. We both tried to show our positive sides while dating like most people do. The fact is that after being married, I got comfortable without always trying to be perfect.

As soon as Mike comes in from work, he asks to see his baby girl, and never asks me how I am doing. This really irritates me as I am his wife. It appears that Mike, my husband is more concerned about his precious child than his wife.

After months of being sick and getting no relief from the meds, I became extremely depressed. It did not appear to me that my husband even cared, as I began to beg him for help in establishing some structure in our family related to my daughter doing her chores, him helping out more in managing the household chores, and for us to spend quality time together as husband and wife and that included going to marriage counseling/therapy.

Mike said no to marital therapy. I went as far as to develop a list of routines to help keep our daughter stay on track and to free me from some of the responsibilities and the constant complaining to her what I needed to be done. Mike said he did not like the list so our daughter never bought into actually completing the chores.

I began to feel a deep isolation as I was too afraid and ashamed to tell my friends what was going on with me. I can remember not answering the telephone when it would ring and I would avoid others by isolating. I had become paranoid. I had three sets of friends: spiritual, religious, and carnal friends. My relationships with all of them were different. I began to question everyone's motives.

Well by May 2014, I could not take it anymore; I was fed up, and angry. I was getting nowhere with the doctors; I was forgetting everything and almost burning the kitchen down. While working from home one day, I had left something on the stove and I had forgotten to check on it.

The stove caught on fire and I ended up having to call 911 and the fire department. I was so embarrassed. I had to tell my employer what had happened. Several similar incidents happened when I had left the bath water running and I had forgotten to turn it off; the water over flowed from the bathroom to the master bedroom carpet. My mind was not functioning properly.

I forgot to mention that I had been in two automobile accidents in September 2013 and then again January 2014 which required me to see a chiropractor due to neck and back injuries. On the mental side of things, I developed post-traumatic stress disorder (PTSD). I also started having panic attacks on a daily basis and did not want to drive my car. I could not drive on the freeway anymore due to fear of getting into another car accident.

All of these issues started impacting every aspect of my life. I was experiencing marital conflicts, parent and child relationship issues and occupational stressors. However, I continued to work in spite of feeling overwhelmed. The work load continued to mount daily, new changes, and more expectations. I found myself working twelve hour days just to get the job done. My relationship with staff/ my peers began to become conflictual and annoying to both them and myself. I found myself completely isolated working from home; be careful what you ask for as you just may get it. I had requested to work from home as I was driving two hours each way. This was very tiring but I did it for three and a half years.

When the opportunity came to start working from home, I jumped for the chance and my supervisor was supportive. I was very excited about not having to commute to work daily; however, the expectation from management was that since I did not have to make the drive and commute, I could easily produce more. Ten percent more was the expectation and I struggled to make the numbers due to my depression, anxiety and now increasing medical conditions.

From January to 2014 to July 2014, I struggled to keep up at work. I found myself becoming very frustrated and disenchanted with everyone. Work stressors was not something new to me as I stated previously, social work can be overwhelming for the most seasoned social workers. If one were to be honest about work stressors, most would say that working in corporate America can be very intense and high pressured work. When you add working in a helping profession where you're clientele have mental illnesses and multiple health problems, the problems become compounded.

If anyone says it's not stressful, I would question their honesty. I know this to be true as I talk with my peers and they all say that the work is stressful. I felt doomed. All the while I was praying for a miracle. I was praying to God that he would fix the situation at work and at home. It appeared, the more I prayed, the worse things became.

My husband went and came as he pleased and did not tell me hello or goodbye. I felt like a stranger and almost a prisoner in my own home. I began to isolate daily and stayed in my room separately from my husband to avoid conflicts with my husband and my daughter. Then the worst things started to happen.

CHAPTER 10
STRONG HOLD AND DEMONIC FORCES

I found myself so angry, so full of rage and resentment not only towards my family, co-workers and friends. I began having disagreements with my friends and found myself feeling hurt and rejected by my friends. They did not seem to understand me and they started avoiding my calls. I had no one to talk to. I decided to start seeing a therapist as at least she would be there to listen. I had previously seen her and she knew my full history so I felt comfortable with her. She told me that my anger, rage and resentment had started way back when I was a little girl six years old being bussed, bullied, and discriminated against. She further told me that the whippings I got were really physical abuse and the teasing and picking on me by my siblings was interpreted by me as being unloved.

As I stated at the beginning of the book, these experiences are based on my own perceptions of how things went down or transpired. I knew that I was angry but I did not think that I had an anger management problem; however, when I began using profanity and growling and grunting like an animal, this was different for me.

I cursed at my daughter and my husband and then I started cursing at people who angered me at the grocery stores, solicitors, telemarketers, and the general public sector. This was so out of character for me. In all the twelve years of my daughter's life, she had never heard me curse nor did my husband. He was so offended and I saw him begin to lose respect for me more and more on a daily basis. He began to avoid me as to avoid an argument. The more he avoided me, the more I would provoke him into an argument.

Being raised in a Pentecostal church; I was familiar with people having the devil in them or demonic possession. I had seen my pastor pray and lay hands on people all of my life, and plead the blood of Jesus for the devil to come out of people. I had been to the doctors and it seemed to me that they were just pumping me with meds and I was not getting any better. Now that I think about it, I felt the meds may have been causing many side effects (the paranoia and the delusional thoughts. The aggressiveness was also concerning for me as I was challenging people twice my size and yelling at them and worst of all cursing people out. I remember while I was on an airplane a huge man was disrespectful to me, I demanded an apology from him and we stared each other down until he said he was sorry.

My friend Shirley (a couple of years older than I) is a very spiritual woman and believes in the gifts and speaking in tongues, prophecy, and "laying hands on the sick." I asked Shirley if she would mind laying hands on me as I felt that I was possessed. She did and I experienced the demonic spirit having warfare within my body and the pull and pressure was so strong that it knocked me down to the ground; I began growling and hollering and screaming. The thought of it today makes me very uncomfortable.

Shirley also had her husband lay hands on me and anoint me with oil. She taught me how to go through my home and put oil and oil crosses on my home for protection. Again I knew how to do some of these things from growing up in the church, but not on a first hand basis. Shirley then told me that I could do this myself and so every time I had that feeling coming up of intense anger, and rage, I would plead the blood of Jesus until the feelings subsided. Then I would get a broom and sweep out the evil spirits out of my house.

Now I know that the intellectual people will say, "Oh she is psychotic and or using religion as a crutch," my response would be "not so." As I am an intelligent woman with a master degree in clinical social work. I know that psychiatry would label this as psychosis, religiosity, grandiose, and paranoia. I know that I have been to the medical professionals and prescribed multiple medications, however, I was still sick; I was still coughing every day and could not stop coughing until I lost my voice. I know that I had stomach issues (IBS) acid reflux disease and a host of other illness that the medications were not curing.

I was going to church and participating in a couple of ministries, but still not really living a faith based life. I had read books, listen to CDS, and DVDS, and heard various preachers preaching on healing, but again I had not experienced this first hand by exercising and practicing faith building exercises. I began really getting into the word and praying for healing. I remember seeing a woman who was a Christian in the grocery store. She stared at me and said she could see the power of the Holy Ghost working in my life as I appeared different to her; she said I had a glow and the spirit of the Lord had told her to tell me that I was beautiful; those kind words meant so much to me as I was really feeling down that day. I didn't have on any make up nor jewelry and that used to be something that I always had to have on before leaving the house.

You see I had become so superficial and materialistic prior to re-dedicating my life to Christ. But now after being sick, I realized that those things were no longer important to me. Actually God revealed this transformation to me as he told me that I did not need all that stuff to make me whole and that he looked at my heart instead of my physical outward appearance. This woman in the grocery store simply re-affirmed God's message to me and there would be subsequent encounters similar to this encounter which continued to show me that God was working in my life.

I stopped listening and watching secular TV for about three to four months, except for Christian channels and programs. I was fed only the word as the news and radio only talked about things that made me more depressed and anxious. For the first time, I really felt close to God in a way like never before. Like I had previously said, I was raised in the church, but it was more of a social experience for me to see my friends and to listen to some good songs. Don't get me wrong, I enjoyed good teaching and or preaching, but I never really let myself "go" in the spirit.

I decided that I needed to visit other churches to venture out where I would receive teachings on the gifts of healing, the power of healing and to develop ways I could get and receive my own healing directly from God and not so much from man. I went to churches, and I went to the prayer lines and asked for healing and the prayer warriors laid hands on me and I felt the anointing of the Lord come over me, and I began to speak in tongues.

Little by little I began to get better. The coughing continued for months I would say about five to six months, but now it was decreasing and generally came on due to stress or allergens from the environment. I continued to listen to my pastor's preaching, TD Jakes, Paula White, Dr. Cindy Trimm, Kenneth Copeland and Charles Stanley, and many others on the gifts of healing, faith, trusting your own instincts (Holy Spirit) and living your true dreams. Joel Olsten was also one of my favourite's; he helped me to stop being so negative. All of the teachings were reinforcing the notions of stop living in the past, stop being a victim, stop trying to change your mate, stop comparing your life with someone else's as everyone has issues. The themes encouraged me to search deep within to find out my true calling and my true destiny.

CHAPTER 11

FORGIVENESS IS THE KEY TO
HAPPINESS

Jesus tells us to forgive as he forgave the people who crucified him. I say I forgive all the people who have wronged me in the past, but have I really? I don't think so or I would not still be having the same feelings of anger and resentment. However, I am continuing to work on forgiving everyone as I really want to live a life freely without anxiety and anger all the time. I now realize that the bondage of not forgiving those that have hurt me was causing physical and mental pain for me. I have told Mike so many times that I forgive him, but he continued to be very distant, cold, and non-communicative. I am wondering if I am just wasting my time trying to re-build a broken marriage.

Sometimes I felt that he really wanted to make our marriage work by the little things he does to show he cares. But I know that it is difficult to live with a person who is an emotional wreck, mood swings, the yelling and the cursing has made him not trust me and distance him even more from me. God tells me to stop worrying about Mike, my marriage, and my relationship with my child and job security. God has told me to just focus on my own healing and let him handle the rest. However, I know that is the best for me, as a social worker, I am a fixer. I am also very analytical so it's difficult for me to "let go and let God." I realize that this is what I should be doing.

I asked two of Mike's friends who just happen to be Christians to talk with him. These men seemed to be strong Christians and appear to have great relationships with their wives. Both men have talked to Mike. They said that Mike has always been very guarded and secretive. His friends also state that Mike came from a very different world than I have and he had to learn to be independent at a young age as he lost his parents at a young age. So actually Mike is also a broken man without the support and guidance of his parents to role model how a husband should really be with his wife. Mike is in denial about his past or perhaps it was so painful for him that he has put up this wall to block any uncomfortable feelings related to his emotions.

We basically avoid each other to avoid arguments. Only God knows the fate of our marriage and I just have to have faith to believe that God will turn things around for us. It will have to take a miracle at this point to mend this broken marriage

At this point, I am not sure when the doctor will say that I am ready to return to work. The demands on the job were so overwhelming. However, God may fix it so that I can continue to work for the same company but in a different position. I am opened to that possibility. I need some rest and I will pray again to God that he will give me some insight or perhaps I will just say yes to your will Lord. I want to do your will whatever that maybe Lord.

CHAPTER 12

GOD HAS SHOWN ME FAVOR

From a material perspective, God blessed me with bill collectors decreasing my medical expenses from a $3000 to $300. Contractors would come to my house and would perform work for me and would not charge me anything;

My husband got a promotion and I was able to receive time off from work as I was recovering from my illnesses. God is so good to me; I was able to keep up with my bills, although I was on disability. When praises went up, blessings came down.

I listened to Kenneth Copeland speak on forgiveness. I can't count the number of times, God has shown me favor. I received checks from companies out of nowhere it appeared. I got an $800 stove for $150. On numerous occasions, I felt God's presence which kept me from getting into car accidents and or pulled over by the police for speeding. Too much information☺

I also felt like God was telling me things in a prophetic way to avoid disaster. My health was starting to improve when God told me to stop seeing my regular PCP and to find another one. My new PCP is a Christian and she actually prescribed medications which were starting to make me feel better. Best of all the coughing has stopped. My sleeping has also started to improve.

While attending a church, the prayer warriors laid hands on people and preached on strong holds and spiritual warfare. I felt Jesus anointing me and I began speaking in tongues something I had not previously experienced as a Christian.

I began going to church and sitting in the front as I wanted to fully appreciate the service and what was being taught. I did not want to hide anymore; I did not want to hold back praising the Lord as the Lord had been so good to me. I praised the Lord with all my might and strength. I raised my hands and truly worshipped the Lord without any reservations. I felt more connected to God than ever before. I spent more time in the word and focusing on scriptures on healing and being grateful. I began trying really hard to please my husband. Cooking him nice meals and complimenting him. I stopped cursing at my husband and my daughter.

I also began to buy him small gifts to show him that I cared. My attitude also began to change towards my daughter. I had neglected her for several months as I was so depressed and could not give her the attention she had been craving. I realize now that the yelling and screaming matches were really her cries out to me for attention and love that she longed for just as I had as a child; but often felt neglected and abandoned by my mother as well.

Now I understand that parenting is not an easy job. My mother could not give me the attention I craved for either as she too was depressed and probably overwhelmed with marital issues just as I was.

CHAPTER 13

I CAN DO ALL THINGS THROUGH CHRIST WHO STRENGTHENS ME.

I just listen to a CD by Kenneth Copeland again on the force of forgiveness. What I learned from his message is that I have to be willing to forgive everyone that has hurt me. That means going all the way back to when I was 7 years old and forgiving those kids who harassed and bullied me.

It also means forgiving the teacher who held me behind one year and the countless boyfriends who broke my heart, and the past co-workers who said I was not management material, and those supervisors who gave me a mediocre review; most importantly, is that I have to forgive my parents, my siblings, and my present family: my husband and my daughter for all the things I wished they would have said or done. If I don't, I will continue to suffer. It's God who tells us we must forgive. I really don't have a choice if I want to be happy and healthy. The recovery process is one step at a time; however, I have to make that first step.

The scales are often unbalanced. Sometimes I give 80% and my husband may give 20 % other times I may give 30 % and my husband may give 70 %. What I have learned from my experiences is that I cannot expect anyone to make me happy. Happiness comes from within a person and not from external things. Living in a big pretty house may be nice, but if you don't have a good relationship with your spouse and child, then what's the point.

I realize also that although I begged the Lord to send me a husband and to have a child, and even though I was 41 years old, I really was not ready emotionally. I realize now that I was so set in my ways and my comfort zone, that I could not share my life with my family freely. I understand now that I had become resentful of having to get up early to make sure our child got off to school. For several years I only had to be concerned with getting myself up and ready for work.

After several weeks of trying to re-build our broken marriage and my getting healthier with prayer, therapy and medication adjustments, I initiated a conversation with my husband regarding us reconciling our marriage. He actually listened to me and we were able to communicate our needs and wants. He shared with me how I had hurt him by avoiding intimacy, and I shared with him the things he had done to hurt me. I asked him to be a support to me in parenting our child and for us to develop structure in our household and to keep the lines of communication open. Little by little, I began to see a change in my husband. We began going to church together again and actually communicating without arguing. My husband began taking out the trash without me asking him. He truly appeared to be trying to improve and be more understanding.

He also initiated organizing our closets, washing his own laundry, buying things for the house, and buying things for me again. He offered to pay for some home repairs and carpet cleaning without me even asking him. His change in behaviors meant a lot to me. Currently, I am counting my blessings. He is helping me by supporting the parenting decisions that I have requested support from him. He also has initiated buying groceries. Now when I talk with him, he actually stops what he is doing to give me his undivided attention and eye contact. Only God has touched my husband's heart and soul to bring about this change. We are still in the process of reconciling our differences, but I have faith that God will bring us through this.

In my humble opinion, to be married is to give up your independence and to become interdependent but not to give up your soul.
I thought that I was ready but I was not. I basically wanted my cake and eat it too. I am not saying that my husband was perfect and that all of our issues were due to my selfishness. No siree, he too is selfish and the two of us together were very stubborn and not willing to compromise.

I decided in order to make my marriage work and to keep our family intact; I would have to be the bigger person. I bought the movie "Fireproof" which is a Christian movie based on the book "Fireproof" and I started doing "The Love Dare" Journal. That was very difficult at first because I would do nice things for Mike, and he would not say "thank you." I just wanted to feel appreciated. Was that asking too much? I think not. It appeared to me he was ungrateful and this really bothered me.

However, in fairness to Mike, I realized he was resentful of me too for being selfish, self centered and non-passionate towards him for all those years. As I stated before, we were both broken which in turn made our marriage broken.

We both made several mistakes in our marriage; however, currently, I am placing God first and taking Sunnie out of the equation. My prayer today is "Lord, let your will be done in our lives." I will no longer try to change my husband as I know that only God can do that. I know that being a good parent means saying "no" at times and being a strong disciplinarian does not necessarily equate to whipping my child.

It has been a long, painful, yet rewarding endeavor. This journey has not always been easy; but I have learned many life lessons from my own experiences and those countless others too many to list here.

ALONG THE WAY, THESE ARE JUST A FEW THAT I HAVE LEARNED:

1. TRUST IN YOUR INSTINCTS.

2. NO WEAPON FORMED AGAINST ME SHALL PROSPER.

3. DON'T TAKE MYSELF AS SERIOUSLY AS NONE ELSE DOES.

4. THE KEY TO HAPPINESS COMES FROM WITHIN AND NOT EXTERNALLY.

5. DON'T COMPARE YOUR LIFE TO OTHERS. YOU HAVE NO IDEA WHAT THEIR JOURNEY IS ALL ABOUT.

6. ENVY IS A WASTE OF TIME. YOU ALREADY HAVE ALL YOU NEED.

7. FORGET ISSUES OF THE PAST.

8. DON'T REMIND YOUR PARTNER ABOUT HIS/HER MISTAKES OF THE PAST.

9. MAKE PEACE WITH YOUR PAST SO IT WON'T SPOIL THE PRESENT.

10. LASTLY, REALIZE THAT LIFE IS A SCHOOL AND WE ARE ALL HERE TO LEARN.

PROBLEMS ARE SIMPLY PART OF THE LIFE LESSONS YOU LEARN WILL LAST A LIFTIME.

God made me back in 1959, and he does not expect me to be perfect so why should I? These and so many lessons have revealed to me this journey is what has made me who I am today. This is "My Journey."

THE END

ABOUT THE AUTHOR

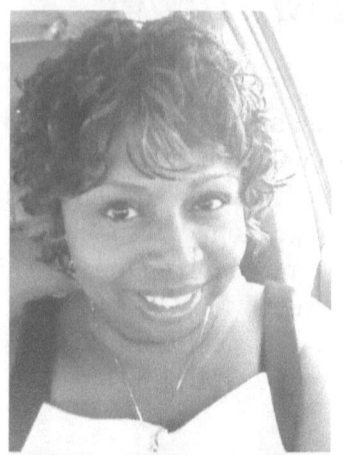

SABRINA RENEE WASHINGTON-POWELL HAS A BACHELOR OF ARTS DEGREE IN SOCIAL SCIENCE, A MASTERDEGREE IN CLINICAL SOCIAL WORK, AND HAS EARNED HER LICENSE IN CLINICAL SOCIAL WORK TO PRACTICE INDEPENDENTLY. SHE HAS WORKED IN THE FIELD OF MENTAL HEALTH FOR APPROXIMATELY THIRTY YEARS. SHE HAS HELD SEVERAL JOBS INCLUDING BUT NOT EXCLUSIVE: PSYCHOTHERAPIST, CASE MANAGER, AND FOSTER FAMILY AGENCY DIRECTOR AND AT HER THE VETERANS ADMINISTRATION HOSPITAL AS A CLINICAL SOCIAL WORKER. SHE HAS BEEN A GUEST SPEAKER ON A TALKLINE SHOW FOR PARENTING AND ANGER MANAGEMENT, SPOKEN AT NATIONAL CONFERENCES ON CULTURAL DIVERSITY AND RACIAL DISPARITIES, AND DEVELOPED CURRICULUM FOR BUILDING SELF- ESTEEM FOR YOUTH. IN HIGH SCHOOL SHE WAS ON THE DEBATE TEAM SHE IS A CHRISTIAN AND ATTENDS CHURCH IN TEXAS. SHE CURRENTLY LIVES IN FORT WORTH TEXAS WITH HER HUSBAND AND THEIR DAUGHTER. DURING HER SPARE TIME, SHE

ENJOYS INTERIOR DECORATING, PHOTOGRAPHY, GARDENING AND ACTING. SHE HAS PORTRAYED MANY CHARACTERS IN LOCAL THEATERS IN FRESNO, CALIFORNIA AND MODESTO, CALIFORNIA.